You Can

Thrive

After Treatment

Also by Debbie Woodbury

How to Build an Amazing Life After Treatment; 10 (more) simple secrets to creating inspired healing, wellness & your joyous life after cancer

You Can
Thrive
After Treatment

10 simple secrets to creating inspired healing, wellness & your joyous life after cancer

Debbie Woodbury

www.WhereWeGoNow.com

For Michael, Emma and Mike.

The reason, the light, and the loves of my life.

You Can Thrive After Treatment

10 simple secrets to creating inspired healing, wellness

& your joyous life after cancer

Disclaimer and FTC Notice

The views expressed are those of the author alone. This book does not provide medical, diagnostic or treatment advice or prescribe the use of any treatment or technique for any physical, emotional or medical problem. The intent of the author is to offer information of a general nature and not to circumvent in any way the advice of a physician. In the event that you use any of the information in this book, you are responsible for your own actions and the author assumes no responsibility therein. Readers may find that websites referred to in this book have changed or disappeared since the book was published.

Your Free Gift

I wrote *The WhereWeGoNow Gratitude Gems Series; Your 30-Day Guide to Jump Starting a Lifetime Gratitude Practice* from a special place of thankfulness. It only seems fitting that I offer it to you as my free gift for buying this book.

If you've been thinking about starting a gratitude practice, or even if it never occurred to you, my guide is easy to follow and fun to read. Each day of the 30-day guide offers an uplifting and inspiring quote, and a Gratitude Practice Tip of the Day to bring an attitude of gratitude into your life.

As a special bonus, the guide also comes with a free download of the *WhereWeGoNow Gratitude Gems* video slideshow. Enjoy three minutes of calming reflection and relaxation. It's sure to make your day!

You can download your free copy of *The WhereWeGoNow Gratitude Gems Series: Your 30-Day Guide to Jump Starting a Lifetime Gratitude Practice* today.[1]

Contents

Preface

A positive attitude is not going to save you. What it's going to do is, every day, between now and the day you die, whether that's a short time from now or a long time from now, that every day, you're going to actually live.
Elizabeth Edwards

Congratulations! You made it to life after treatment! Testing, getting a diagnosis, radiation, chemotherapy, surgeries, recuperation - it's behind you. You should be ecstatic, but something is not quite right.

Instead, you're bone-tired, angry, lost, lonely, stressed, afraid, abandoned and confused. You're keenly aware and scared of possible recurrence.

You don't see your health professionals on a weekly basis anymore. Your family and friends are desperate to put cancer behind them. You'd love to do that too, but you're only just beginning to understand the emotional fallout of living with cancer.

The hard truth is that surviving isn't easy. After I was diagnosed with breast cancer and had a mastectomy, I met with a therapist to work through the emotional issues of my survival. I remember an especially painful session in which I confessed that "living is hard too."

That period was one of the most difficult of my life. It took time, but I hung in there, did the work and slowly discovered 20 secrets to creating inspired healing, wellness and live out loud joy after cancer. (Yes, I said 20. This book is the first in the After Treatment series. The second book in the series is *How to Build an Amazing Life After Treatment; 10 (more) simple secrets to creating inspired healing, wellness & your joyous life after cancer.*[2]

I suggest you use this book like a guide or workbook. Start by reading it through, taking your time – the last thing I want is for you to feel overwhelmed. After you finish the book, go back and focus on the secret or secrets that speak to you. If you're up for making changes, begin with something that comes easily and build up your confidence from there.

Let's start off with a bonus secret: Having a positive attitude doesn't require over-the-top, Pollyanna optimism. What it requires is basking in the glimmer of hope offered by my 20 secrets.

I know *You Can Thrive After Treatment* because I'm doing it. Now I want to help you thrive too. Let's get started creating your inspired healing, wellness and joyous life now.

Secret No. 1

Show Up To Be Supported

Part of the healing process is sharing with other people who care.
Jerry Cantrell

"Show up to be supported" is hands down the number one secret to creating inspired healing, wellness and live out loud joy after cancer.

I know because I went six and a half months from mammogram to mastectomy without support. Sure, I had family and friends who did their absolute best to be there for me. But, they were just as helpless and frightened as I was, and they couldn't possibly understand what I was going through.

Finally, I found the support of medical professionals and other survivors who "got it." In a split second, I went from a feeling of drowning to grabbing onto a vital lifeline that saved me.

Do you feel alone and angry that no one really gets what you've been through and what you're still struggling with as a cancer survivor? Wouldn't it be great to get the emotional support you need and deserve?

I've got two words of advice for you: **Show up!**

During that first six and one half months of my cancer experience, I did nothing to get support. This was despite the fact that I knew about organizations that would have taken me in with open arms. I didn't contact them because I didn't know all I had to do was show up.

Once I grabbed hold of the lifeline of support, I learned important truths. I had to show up. I had to share (when I was ready.) I had to be vulnerable. I had to hear others, even when their stories scared me. I had to feel the pain and let it move through me. I had to trust.

Because I started showing up, amazing people came into my life and formed my circle of support, including my nurse navigator, oncology therapist, rehabilitation exercise therapist, massage therapist and all of the fellow survivors I've met personally and through my website, www.WhereWeGoNow.com

I recently spoke at a survivorship symposium where a man approached me with a shy smile. He hesitantly told me about his wife's oral cancer and how he was taking care of her. I asked who was supporting him and he answered "No one" with tears in his eyes. Of course, that made my eyes well with tears too.

We talked about why it was vital to get individual support for him and his wife, and how they were both in pain and unable to fully support the other alone.

Despite his shyness, that man bravely walked up to me. Because he did that, I heard him, related to his pain and connected him with support services at the cancer center.

No one can do cancer alone. Every survivor needs the support of others who "get it." Show up at support groups, make an appointment with a therapist, call cancer help lines and seek out professionals who support your physical, mental and emotional healing. We all need to be supported and support is out there for you if you have the courage to show up.

To get you started, here are a few organizations that you can reach out to for support:

American Cancer Society[3] - Learn about making treatment decisions, coping with side effects, handling financial matters, caregiving, and living well after cancer. The ACS also has programs and services to help you manage cancer treatment and recovery and find the emotional support you need. All of their services are free.

Cancer Care[4] – Speak for free with an oncology social worker trained to provide you with support, information and resources to help you and your loved ones better cope with cancer.

Cancer Hope Network[5] – Offering free and confidential one-on-one support to cancer patients and their families. CHN matches cancer patients and their family members with trained volunteers who have undergone and recovered from similar cancer experiences. I'm a support volunteer with this amazing organization. Maybe we'll be a match!

Cancer Support Community[6] - Whether you are newly diagnosed with cancer or a long-time cancer survivor, caring for someone with cancer, or a health care professional looking for resources, the CSC's toll-free Cancer Support Helpline is available to you Monday through Friday, 9 am- 8 pm EST.

Livestrong Foundation[7] - Provides free, confidential one-on-one support in English and Spanish to anyone with cancer or to loved ones, friends, health care professionals or caregivers.

Secret No. 2

Tell Your Story

There is no greater agony than bearing an untold story inside you.
Maya Angelou

You can show up for support, never open your mouth and reap benefits. If you really want to ramp up your healing, however, you should consider telling your story.

We all have a story. No, let me rephrase that: We all have stories. As cancer survivors, we have diagnostic stories, treatment stories, doctor stories, family and friends stories, survivorship stories - the list goes on and on. There is no end to the stories, but what we might not have is the ability to tell our stories.

And let's be honest. The further we get down the survivorship road, the less and less time we are allotted to share our cancer stories. Once others in our lives have returned to normal, they aren't as likely to be willing listeners. You can't really blame them, but what do we do with our stories?

The answer is personal to the individual. When I first discovered the world of cancer support services, I tried joining support groups and one-on-one therapy. I found that I shared the most with my therapist, but still attended support groups to be with other survivors.

Now, I tell my story by blogging[8], tweeting,[9] and sharing on Facebook.[10] When I need to share more privately, I turn to the group of survivor-friends I have gathered around me.

For others, there is journaling or keeping a diary. Putting pen to paper or fingers to keyboard, unleashes emotional and physical catharsis. The beauty of journaling is the release of our untold story into a space of safety and total privacy. When journaling, you can write anything you want, without fear of offense or reprisal.

Art, and specifically drawing, is another compelling way to release the story within. At a recent survivors' symposium we were invited to draw to music by an art therapist. A friend and I worked together and fell into a discussion about our scars. We shared their location, how we got them and, most importantly, how we felt about them. It was an amazing moment of telling our "scar stories."

I believe self-expression and validation are at the heart of support. Being heard allows us to work through our emotional issues and helps us heal. Speak up at your support group, talk with a therapist, or pick up a pen, a musical instrument, paint brush or lump of clay. Tell your untold story in whatever way feels natural to you.

Secret No. 3

Practice Gratitude

At times our own light goes out and is rekindled by a spark from another person. Each of us has cause to think with deep gratitude of those who have lighted the flame within us.
Albert Schweitzer

You were run over by the cancer bus but, if you're alive and have the support you deserve, there are lots of reasons to say "thank you!" Once I found support as a cancer survivor, overwhelming gratitude for each of my supporter's unique gifts of healing replaced fear as my primary emotion.

As I healed from my diagnosis, mastectomy and reconstructive surgeries, it was gratitude that pulled me up and through the emotional turmoil. It was gratitude that revealed the gifts of cancer[11] and helped me absorb the losses. It was gratitude that inspired me to create a community of survivors sharing our new normal lives after cancer.

Gratitude also made me a compulsive thank you letter writer. I'm not talking about polite thank you notes written from social obligation. Oh no, I'm talking about raw, openly emotional missives from the heart. I had to let these very special people know I couldn't have done it without them.

Probably because they came from the heart, these letters always made me feel vulnerable and I usually put off sending them for days after they were written. To a person, however, the response was always kind, appreciative and truly touching. What really struck me was how happy they were to hear from me, which I really never expected.

I also never expected my little thank you notes to have big effects. One email I wrote was to a very special medical professional who gave me incredible support and guidance. She responded, telling me how happy she was to hear from me, especially as she was now struggling with career decisions.

A few weeks later she sent me another email saying it was her turn to thank me. My earlier email had helped her crystalize what she loved doing and she set about getting back to it. Now, she was happy to report that she was back on track and happily pursuing her passion.

Her email brought tears to my eyes. Before I sent my email, I struggled with insecurity and was uncomfortable reaching out to her. Now, she was thanking me for inspiring her to follow her heart and find joy again in her career. My gratitude had come full circle.

Is there someone who made a real difference in your healing? Have you told them how much they mean to you? The most beautiful gratitude practice is also the simplest:

If the only prayer you ever say in your entire life is thank you, it will be enough. Meister Eckhart

To help get you started strengthening your attitude of gratitude, make sure to sign up[12] for your free gift, *The WhereWeGoNow Gratitude Gems Series: Your 30-Day Guide to Jump Starting a Lifetime Gratitude Practice.*

Secret No. 4

Give Back

I have found that among its other benefits, giving
liberates the soul of the giver.
Maya Angelou

One of the secrets of life is that all that is really worth the doing is
what we do for others.
Lewis Carroll

I remember the exact moment I discovered cancer support services. I was lying in my hospital bed, two days after my mastectomy and reconstructive surgery. I was emotional. Heck, the truth is I was a complete mess.

My nurses were heroically trying to console me, but I was having none of it. The reality of my situation had come crashing down on me. I couldn't believe I was there six and a half months after that first suspicious mammogram, lying in a hospital bed completely disabled and minus a body part. Worse, I pictured myself discharged, returning home to face my physical, mental and emotional recuperation alone.

Suddenly another nurse walked into the room and introduced herself as my nurse navigator. She sat beside my bed and calmly let me know I was not alone. She and the cancer support services offered at my cancer center were there to support me on every level now and after I returned home.

In that moment I went from drowning in hopelessness to grabbing onto a vital lifeline that saved me. I left the hospital and began showing up for every sort of support service I could and, in the beginning, all I could manage in return was a heartfelt "thank you."

As I progressed, I needed to do more than simply express my gratitude in words. I needed to give back. Opportunities fell into my lap – encouraging other survivors, volunteering with the Cancer Hope Network,[13] working as a patient educator with the Pathways Women's Cancer Teaching Project[14] and creating www.WhereWeGoNow.com, to name just a few.

I know how it feels to be worn out with no energy for anything other than keeping yourself going. No one expects you to throw yourself into volunteer work right after you finish chemo. Take your time, heal, and, if you're interested, opportunities will come your way when you are up to them.

In the meantime, every time you look into another patient's eyes and tell her you "get it," please know that you are giving back in the most meaningful way possible.

The first time I gave back[15] it was in service to another survivor. As we spoke, I felt something I had never thought was possible – my cancer experience was actually useful, because it was pressed into service to a fellow survivor. In that moment my soul was liberated from cancer's grip and it was the beginning of the end of my cancer depression.

As we express our gratitude, we must never forget that the highest appreciation is not to utter words, but to live by them. John F. Kennedy

Secret No. 5

Honor Your Anger

Bitterness is like cancer. It eats upon the host.
But anger is like fire. It burns it all clean.
Maya Angelou

It's a struggle, but you're working on healing. You're showing up for support, telling your story, expressing your gratitude, and giving back. So why are you still carrying around the hot, burning ember of cancer anger?

The fact is that anger is merely an emotion – a conscious mental reaction of the psyche to a specific situation or set of facts. It is neither negative nor positive.

Unfortunately, we often consider anger to be a negative and try to avoid it at all costs. The social message is loud and clear: Don't overreact, don't yell, don't curse, don't scream, and don't ever be impolite. Hold it in at all cost. But how do we cope with cancer anger?

As a cancer survivor, I remember a lot to be angry about. Although I never wondered "why me," I did feel anger about changes to my body, loneliness, and having to deal with past emotional traumas stirred up by cancer. I was especially angry when a year had passed since my diagnosis and I was not yet "over" cancer.

I also remember being really angry at the people who wanted to move on and forget about my cancer before I was ready to do the same. I felt alone, abandoned and unheard. As my anger increased, it got too big to share with those same people. The only thing that saved me was being able to voice my anger to my therapist. I know it is only due to her being there for me that I was able to work through my cancer anger[16] and get to a better place in those relationships.

The first mammogram I had after my surgeries caused boatloads of anger. I was already emotional about returning to the scene of my initial bad news, but the technician's insensitivity pushed me over the edge. She started off on the wrong foot by talking about my history in the middle of the waiting room, where our conversation could be overheard.

In the dressing room, she asked me again about my history (she couldn't seem to understand why I only needed a mammogram of my left breast.) Finally, I realized she didn't believe that I had had a mastectomy, despite the fact that I told her so many times. At that point, she told me that many patients don't always know the difference between a lumpectomy and a mastectomy. Really? You try having a mastectomy and then tell me you don't know the difference.

Next, she moved on to my diagnosis, which in her opinion (despite her lack of a medical degree), was "not breast cancer." This shocked me, but I looked her straight in the eye and responded that it was in fact cancer. Not to be deterred, she responded by saying that there was some debate whether it was or wasn't. At that point, I stopped talking because I didn't want to break down and cry, or possibly punch her.

Despite my silence, she kept talking. She told me she knew someone else who had DCIS and she had a mastectomy too, "so she wouldn't have to worry about it anymore." Could she not sense my intense worry and upset at that very moment? Or did she actually think that my mastectomy made it all better and I had nothing to worry about anymore?

When the mammogram was completed, she invited me to take a rose. I considered not taking it, because I was nauseous from the whole experience, but I did to keep my head down. I got dressed, holding myself together, walked as fast as I could out to my car, where I broke down and cried. When I got home, I threw away the rose.

A day later, I was still over the top angry and knew I had to honor my anger. I decided to call the breast center and complain. When I talked about it later with my therapist, she applauded me for calling, but asked why I felt I had to hold it all in while I was there, rather than let the technician see the hurt she had caused. It was an excellent question.

The bitterness of cancer anger was exactly what I was feeling before I made that phone call. By holding it in, I caused it to eat through me, rather than use it to deal with the source of the problem. Once I honored my anger (by acting on it in a constructive way) it burned clean my resentment and bitterness. I felt validated. I felt empowered and I felt heard.

Are you experiencing cancer anger? If so, please know that it's normal and you are more than entitled to it. Just remember that it's okay to express your anger, especially when you do so constructively before it builds up to tragic proportions.

Secret No. 6

Move Your Body

If any thing is sacred, the human body is sacred.
Walt Whitman

Before cancer, I had no use for regular exercise. It's not that I hadn't tried, but I just couldn't get into the routine of going to the gym. I also had bad memories of aerobic exercise classes in which I felt spastic and completely lost.

Of course, my two cancer surgeries took a major toll on my body. I was desperate to do something to improve my body image so I dove back in and joined the local Y. Given my fear of aerobic exercise classes, I started using the weight room, something I had never done before in my life. I was committed and went regularly, but I could feel my interest waning fast. So, I tried a Pilate's class.

The class was crowded and I was lying on my mat in the middle of the floor. It was going okay until the instructor told us to lie on our backs and raise our feet off the ground. My feet would not budge. Not an inch, not a half inch. Not to make excuses, but my TRAM flap reconstruction had me down to one transverse rectus abdominis muscle where there used to be two. Plus, I was totally out of shape.

Of course, that's the intellectual response. I actually responded with shame and total abject grief. I was shocked to find yet another cancer loss - the ability to do something so seemingly simple. I wanted to run out of the room weeping, but was stopped by a vision of trampling other women who could lift their feet off the floor.

Pilates wasn't for me. I had thought about doing yoga before my diagnosis, but didn't make the time. Now, I sought out a beginner's class which sounded perfect: "Stress Management Yoga." Before class began, the teacher welcomed and reassured me that yoga was noncompetitive and wherever I was in my abilities was exactly where I was supposed to be at that moment. I followed along as best I could and it was love at first down dog.

A few months after that first class, I attempted the boat pose and my feet miraculously went straight up in the air. I had tried it before and couldn't do it, so I was stunned. I've come a long way from that Pilates class and discovering yoga brought me there.

Find physical activities that honor your body and tap into that sacred place where you are today. Moving your body will help you take back control, reduce stress and improve body image. Take it a little at a time, but get moving now!

Secret No. 7

Embrace Change

Action and reaction, ebb and flow, trial and error, change - this is the rhythm of living. Out of our over-confidence, fear; out of our fear, clearer vision, fresh hope. And out of hope, progress.
Bruce Barton

"Reinvention" is a euphemism for a much blunter word that scares many of us. That word is "change."

It's easy to hate change. We cringe, gulp, deny and fight it every step of the way. Rather than accept it as the only true constant in life, we perceive it as foreign and unsettling. "Change" has a bad reputation.

Let's try to break free of this mind-set. Let's embrace the word "change" and its positive cousin, "reinvention" by looking at change through different eyes:

1. **Without change, something sleeps inside us, and seldom awakens. The sleeper must awaken. Frank Herbert** - Change wakes us up and makes us re-evaluate our priorities and choices.

2. **You must be the change you wish to see in the world. Mahatma Gandhi** - Change isn't only something that happens to us, we can and must be proactive if we want to make change for the better in the world.

3. **If you don't like something change it. If you can't change it, change your attitude. Maya Angelou** - If you are enduring difficulties, you always have a choice as to how you approach your situation.

4. **Change your life today. Don't gamble on the future, act now, without delay. Simone de Beauvoir** - So many of us put off making changes out of fear of the unknown. The bottom line is all we have is today. If you want to make a change, do it now.

5. **Life is about not knowing, having to change, taking the moment and making the best of it, without knowing what's going to happen next. Gilda Radner** - Gilda faced terminal cancer and came to embrace life as "delicious ambiguity." Her book, *It's Always Something*,[17] is one of the first I read after my diagnosis and her ability to face change and the fear it brought will always inspire me.

6. **If you realize that all things change, there is nothing you will try to hold on to. If you are not afraid of dying, there is nothing you cannot achieve. Lao Tzu -** We fear change because of the pain it can cause. Think of what you could achieve if you relinquished that fear through acceptance.

7. **Every great dream begins with a dreamer. Always remember, you have within you the strength, the patience, and the passion to reach for the stars to change the world. Harriet Tubman** - Amen!

I think facing change will always be a bit scary, because most of us aren't fans of the unknown. If your "new normal" life is scaring you, be extra kind to yourself. Remember that you're not alone, especially if you're showing up for support. We're here for each other!

Secret No. 8

Watch Your Breath

Quite simply, if you're feeling anxious, angry, a sense of shame, whatever it is, breathe in and agree to touch or feel it. Breathing out, offer space and care to whatever's there. If there's blocking to touching it, emphasize the in-breath and stay embodied.
Tara Brach

Remember those days when your brain was hijacked by cancer? Every thought you had, at every waking moment, centered on cancer. When I went to bed at night I fought for sleep through a barrage of cancer thoughts. When I awoke, I resisted consciousness because it meant diving back into constant cancer chatter.

Once the days of cancer diagnosis and treatment waned, my ultimate goal was to return to a "normal" existence. But since cancer, I've learned that my "normal" multi-tasking thoughts are no better for my psyche than single-minded anxiety. The best tool I've found to reduce stress in my "new normal" life is the ability to watch my breath.

Watching your breath is the first step to increased mindfulness and awareness. It's also the foundation of meditation. You can practice just minutes a day and, before you know it, you will turn to watching your breath without thinking whenever life gets hectic.

When I wanted to learn to meditate, I turned to *8 Minute Meditation –Quiet Your Mind, Change Your Life*,[18] by Victor Davich. This book makes it easy to get started:

1. Find a comfortable position, upright, but not tense.
2. Set a timer for a few minutes – five to eight minutes works well in the beginning.
3. Close your eyes.
4. Notice your breath, if forced, let it relax.
5. When thoughts enter your mind, notice them, but don't attach to them. There is no need to figure anything out; just let your thoughts float by like clouds in the sky.
6. Continue to follow the breath, in and out. Whenever you leave the breath to follow a thought, and you will, just return to it and try again.

Watching your breath is the single best way to deal with anxiety. It's simple, easy, free and can be done anywhere, at any time. Remember to give it a try next time you're at your oncologist's office, or just sitting in traffic. Knowing how to watch your breath is a gift.

Secret No. 9

Practice Mindfulness

We tend to think of meditation in only one way.
But life itself is a meditation.
Raul Julia

The more I practice mindful awareness, the more I learn what it is and what it isn't. It is not hours spent in the lotus position, eyes closed, blissfully deep in meditation.

I discovered what it is quite by accident when I lost my glasses.

I wear and don't wear glasses. What I mean is that I have them off as often as I have them on. When they're not perched on my nose, I usually have no idea where they are. That's because I mindlessly put them down and, when I want to perch them on my nose again, have no memory of where I put them.

Mindfulness is the opposite of "mind fullness." It's the ability to focus on exactly what is happening at the moment - even something so little as taking off my glasses. Although multi-tasking seems productive in theory, it has repercussions. Like losing your glasses again and again and again. Lose them often enough and it's a short leap from losing your glasses to losing your mind.

Losing my glasses taught me that mindfulness is about conscious awareness of the little things in life. For example:

1. **Glasses** - We all know it's not about the glasses. It's about juggling 20 things at a time. By slowing down and concentrating on one activity we instill calmness and focus. When I let myself single task, I actually get more done with less downtime, because I don't do silly things like constantly losing my glasses.

2. **Yoga and Exercise** - I hit the yoga mat after running out of the house, driving through traffic and running up to class. Sometimes (okay, most times) it's not easy to leave the fury of the day behind and settle into yoga. But when I do, even for a few minutes, I am richly rewarded. That's why I keep going back.

3. **Cooking -** At the end of a busy day, cooking can be a chore, but when you "throw it on the table," you're missing an opportunity for mindfulness. Slow down and really look at your ingredients. Focus on the smell, taste and feel of the food in your hands. Bringing together even a simple dish is a work of creation. Mindfully enjoy it and cooking becomes a relaxing focal point to the day.

4. **Eating -** Once you've mindfully created dinner, why not mindfully eat it? The secret to filling your life with simple pleasures (and food has to be right up there) is to actually pay attention to them. Eat slowly and really taste your food. Your body deserves to be fed and your consciousness deserves to savor it.

5. **Conversation -** Whether it's dinnertime with the family or throughout the day, good conversation requires mindfulness. Do you know that flow that comes when you're talking with a friend and time flies by? That's mindfulness and it's amazing. Resolve to get more of it by mindfully focusing on the person you're talking to at the moment.

6. **Simple Tasks -** When I was a young lawyer, I lived in an apartment by myself for a few years. At the end of my very long, crazy days, I'd find myself washing the dishes and really enjoying it. It was quiet, the soap and warm water relaxed me and I was able to start and finish a project. (If you've ever had a job where nothing ever seems to resolve or be finished, you know what I mean.) I didn't know what mindfulness was at the time, but that's what I was experiencing and it was very satisfying.

7. **Relaxation –** Relaxing doesn't come easily to me, but I know I need to refresh and rejuvenate more often. Being mindfully connected to the moment of relaxation (and not running unending to-do lists through my head) is my only hope. I'm working on it.

8. **Sex -** See #7 and read more about how to "Spice Up Your Sex Life," which is Secret No. 7 in my second book of the After Treatment series, *How to Build an Amazing Life After Treatment; 10 (more) simple secrets to creating inspired healing, wellness & your joyous life after cancer.*[19]

9. **Tea meditation -** It's funny how a little thing like tea can teach so much about mindfulness.[20]

10. **Silence -** How can we be mindfully aware of any one thing with so many distractions constantly swirling around us? With all of our 24/7 gadgetry, we've forgotten that moments of silence are necessities. Resolve to turn off the unnecessary noise in your day and seek out silence (or as close to silence as you can get.) Making moments of silence a priority makes mindfulness a possibility.

The most important thing to realize about mindfulness is how focusing on the present keeps you from obsessing about the future. When we are mindful, we're not worrying about future events that may or may not happen and making ourselves anxious. Mindfulness quiets the mind, helps us relax and heal, and taps into our inner strength.

Secret No. 10

Sleep Better

Sleep is the best meditation.
Dalai Lama

Living the hectic, stressful lives we live, we often forget how to push the "Off" button. We work, run from place to place, and are anxiety ridden to distraction. We're cancer survivors who power up each morning, because we have a lot to do and we're so grateful for the ability to do it. Yet, we might not be as good at powering down at night and getting the rest we need to support our full lives after cancer.

A few months after my mastectomy, I met an exercise instructor at a support group. She was very upset that breast cancer kept her from exercising. Finally, her doctor cleared her to exercise and she threw herself back into it with a vengeance. Now she was in a lot of pain, mad at the doctor and afraid she could never return to what she loved. As we talked, it became obvious she had the drive to return to exercising once she let herself heal. What she wasn't able to do was relax.

It's hard to relax when our minds are in turmoil. But without relaxation we can't get the sleep we need to recharge and focus productively. If you're finding it hard to get to sleep, follow my ten tips to help you get the sleep you need:

1. **Set a regular bedtime and time to get up each morning**. Follow through on the weekends. A regular sleep schedule will help ease you into the routine of good sleep.

2. **Have quiet time before bedtime.** Avoid television, smartphone and computer screens, because the light they throw off is a stimulant.[21] Plus, how many times have you watched a particularly violent episode of a TV show, or been disturbed by the news? Let only good thoughts come your way before going to bed.

3. **Make sure your bedroom is dark, cool and quiet.**

4. **Don't drink alcohol, caffeinated beverages, or eat or drink too much before bedtime.** Caffeine is a stimulant and, although alcohol may initially make you sleepy, it may also act as a stimulant[22] and you will find yourself wide awake a few hours later. As for other liquids, no one likes to make frequent trips to the bathroom when they should be sleeping.

5. **If you still can't get to sleep after about 15 minutes of trying, focus on relaxation, rather than sleep.** The more we focus on not sleeping the more likely we are to create insomnia.

6. **Listen to guided imagery or calming music on your iPod while comfortably lying in bed.** I started doing this before I had my mastectomy[23] because my anxiety was keeping me up at night. It usually worked wonders and still does.

7. **Journaling or writing is a calming activity when you can't sleep.** Putting your anxieties and worries down on paper may be all you need to do at 3 a.m. to feel more in control of the situation. If you

are awake because your head is full of ideas, write them down. Visualize the ideas out of your head and on the paper, where they can sit and wait for you to get back to them tomorrow.

8. **Drink herbal tea and honey and curl up in a blanket.** A little bit of TLC in the middle of the night goes a long way to making you feel more relaxed and nurtured.

9. **Listen to the silence, really hear it.** The middle of the night is like no other time of the day (especially if you have a busy job, family life, etc.) Sometimes I realize I'm awake because I need to hear silence.[24]

10. **Breathe and practice mindfulness during the day.** If we practice mindfulness during the day, we will be that much better at quieting the "what if's?" at night. Anyone who has ever dealt with insomnia knows that the more upset you get about it, the more likely you are to stay awake. Mindfulness keeps you from panicking, and that may be all you need to eventually get yourself to sleep.

Give yourself the gift of mindfulness and breathing during the day, and it will reward you with the best meditation during the night. I hope you get a good night's rest!

WhereWeGoNow

From Here

I always remind myself that "simple doesn't mean easy." You and I know all too well that it's not easy to thrive after cancer and this book doesn't offer any magic potions around that fact.

What I hope you get from this book are simple ways to rebuild your life after cancer, support from someone who's been where you are, and hope that you too can thrive after cancer.

The bottom line is that thriving takes patience. As you begin the process of going from active treatment to creating a life after cancer, it might feel as if you are slogging through oatmeal. Despite that very real feeling, you really are moving forward and, eventually, you will see progress.

Hang in there and take each day as it comes.

I'm honored and thrilled to be a part of your journey and would love to keep our conversation going. Join me at www.WhereWeGoNow.com

and make sure to sign up to receive updates, information and free downloads.

If you've found You Can Thrive After Treatment encouraging, make sure to check out the second book in the After Treatment series - *How to Build an Amazing Life after Treatment; 10 (more) simple secrets to creating inspired healing, wellness & your joyous life after cancer.*[25]

As you work through my ten simple secrets and explore where you go now from here, keep this in mind:

Do the one thing you think you cannot do. Fail at it. Try again. Do better the second time. The only people who never tumble are those who never mount the high wire. This is your moment. Own it. Oprah Winfrey

This is your moment to take that first step to be supported, tell your story, practice gratitude, give back, honor your anger, love your body, embrace change, watch your breath, practice mindfulness and sleep better.

It's up to you to decide what your life after cancer will look like and I'm proud to support your efforts.

You can do this.

Thank You

I can't tell you enough how much I appreciate your taking the time to read my book. Writing this book was a labor of love and it is an honor to share it with you.

If you enjoyed the book and found it helpful, please consider leaving a review on Amazon. Having reviews of this book on Amazon is essential to getting it found by people who could benefit from reading it. For that reason, every review really helps and I would be eternally grateful to you for taking the time to write one for me.

To leave a review, all you need to do is go to the review section on the book's Amazon page. Click the button that says "Write a customer review"[26] and you're off!

Thank you again for your support and I wish you all the best as you create inspired healing, wellness and your joyous life after cancer!

Survival > Existence,

Debbie

www.WhereWeGoNow.com

P.S. – Don't forget to collect my special thank you free gift. If you haven't done so already, download *The WhereWeGoNow Gratitude Gems Series: Your 30-Day Guide to Jump Starting a Lifetime Gratitude Practice* today.[27]

About Debbie

Maya Angelou said, *"There is no greater agony than bearing an untold story inside you."* The healing power of sharing her story compelled Debbie to found www.WhereWeGoNow.com, a community for cancer survivors creating inspired healing, wellness and live out loud joy. She is also a blogger at The Huffington Post,[28] an inspirational speaker, a support volunteer with The Cancer Hope Network,[29] a member of the Carol G. Simon Cancer Center Oncology Community Advisory Board, a patient educator with the Pathways Women's Cancer Teaching Project,[30] a wife and mother, and a former very stressed out lawyer.

Debbie has been quoted by Cure Magazine on survivorship issues in *Survivor Defined*[31] and *Seeing Red: Coping with Anger During Cancer.*[32]

Debbie is also the author of *How to Build an Amazing Life After Treatment; 10 (more) simple secrets to creating inspired healing, wellness & your joyous life after cancer.*[33]

You can also find Debbie on Twitter[34] and Facebook.[35]

Notes

[1]Sign up form, *The WhereWeGoNow Gratitude Gems Series: Your 30-Day Guide to Jump Starting a Lifetime Gratitude Practice*. Web. 1 Nov. 2013. <http://wherewegonow.us2.listmanage.com/subscribe?u=915e27d7085c84e5a4a24e f74&id=db818ecfb0>.

[2] Woodbury, Debbie. *How to Build an Amazing Life After Treatment*, WhereWeGoNow, LLC, 2013.<http://www.amazon.com/Build-Amazing-After-Treatment-ebook/dp/B00G60UBLQ>.

[3] *American Cancer Society, Find Support and Treatment*, Web. 1 Nov. 2013. <http://www.cancer.org/treatment/index >.

[4]*Cancer Care*, Web. 1 Nov. 2013. <http://www.cancercare.org>.

[5]*Cancer Hope Network*, Web. 1 Nov. 2013. <http://www.cancerhopenetwork.org>.

[6] *Cancer Support Community*, Web. 1 Nov. 2013. <http://www.cancersupportcommunity.org/MainMenu/Cancer-Support/Cancer-Support-Helpline.html>.

[7] *Livestrong*, Web. 1 Nov. 2013. <http://intakes.livestrong.org/cancersupport/>.

[8] Woodbury, Debbie, Blog Archive, *WhereWeGoNow*, WhereWeGoNow LLC, Web. 1 Nov. 2013. <http://www.wherewegonow.com/blog>.

[9] Woodbury, Debbie on Twitter @DebbieWWGN, Web. 1 Nov. 2013. <https://twitter.com/DebbieWWGN>.

[10] WhereWeGoNow as Cancer Survivors, Facebook page. Web. 1 Nov. 2013. <https://facebook.com/pages/WhereWeGoNow-As-Cancer-Survivors/197760313589739>.

[11] Woodbury, Debbie, *WhereWeGoNow*, Debbie's Gifts & Losses List, *WhereWeGoNow*, WhereWeGoNow LLC, Web. 1 Nov. 2013. <http://www.wherewegonow.com/gifts-and-losses/debbies-list>.

[12] Sign up form, *The WhereWeGoNow Gratitude Gems Series: Your 30-Day Guide to Jump Starting a Lifetime Gratitude Practice*. Web. 1 Nov. 2013. <http://wherewegonow.us2.listmanage.com/subscribe?u=915e27d7085c84e5a4a24e f74&id=db818ecfb0>.

[13] *Cancer Hope Network*, Web. 1 Nov. 2013. <http://www.cancerhopenetwork.org>.

[14] *Pathways Women's Cancer Teaching Project*. Web. 1 Nov. 2013.
<http://womenscancerteachingproject.org/>.

[15] Woodbury, Debbie. "Coming out of Cancer Depression: Giving Back by
Supporting Others Helps Me Heal Too" Weblog post. *WhereWeGoNow*,
WhereWeGoNow, LLC, Web. 1 Nov. 2013.
<http://www.wherewegonow.com/debbies-blog/coming-out-cancer-depression-
giving-back-supporting-others-helps-me-heal-too>.

[16] Woodbury, Debbie. "Do You Share Your Bad Attitude Toward Cancer?" Weblog
post. *WhereWeGoNow*, WhereWeGoNow, LLC, Web. 1 Nov. 2013.
<http://www.wherewegonow.com/debbies-blog/do-you-share-your-bad-attitude-
toward-cancer>.

[17] Radner, Gilda. *It's Always Something*. Sydney: Simon and Schuster, 1989. Print.

[18] Davich, Victor N. *8 Minute Meditation: Quiet Your Mind, Change Your Life*. New York:
Perigee, 2004. Print.

[19] Woodbury, Debbie. How to Build an Amazing Life After Treatment,
WhereWeGoNow, LLC, 2013. <http://www.amazon.com/Build-Amazing-After-
Treatment-ebook/dp/B00G60UBLQ>.

[20] Woodbury, Debbie. "Have You Stopped for Tea Meditation Today?" Weblog post.
WhereWeGoNow, WhereWeGoNow, LLC, Web. 1 Nov.. 2013.
<http://www.wherewegonow.com/debbies-blog/have-you-stopped-tea-meditation-
today>.

[21] O'Connor, Anahad. "Really? Using a Computer Before Bed Can Disrupt Sleep."
Weblog post. *New York Times*. New York Times, 10 Sept. 2012. Web. 1 Nov. 2013.
<http://well.blogs.nytimes.com/2012/09/10/really-using-a-computer-before-bed-
can-disrupt-sleep/?_r=2>.

[22] "Twelve Simple Tips to Improve Your Sleep." Web log post. *Healthy Sleep*. Division
of Sleep Medicine at Harvard Medical School, 18 Dec. 2007. Web. 1 Nov. 2013.
<http://healthysleep.med.harvard.edu/healthy/getting/overcoming/tips>.

[23] Woodbury, Debbie. "Orange Day Lilies & Surgery, Perfect Together" Weblog post.
WhereWeGoNow, WhereWeGoNow, LLC, Web. 1 Nov. 2013.
<http://www.wherewegonow.com/debbies-blog/orange-day-lilies-surgery-perfect-
together.>

[24] Woodbury, Debbie, "Meditation Monday – The Necessity of Silence in Our Lives."
Weblog post. *WhereWeGoNow*, WhereWeGoNow LLC, Web. 1 Nov. 2013.
<http://www.wherewegonow.com/debbies-blog/meditation-monday-necessity-
silence-our-lives>.

[25] Woodbury, Debbie. *How to Build an Amazing Life After Treatment*, WhereWeGoNow, LLC, 2013. <http://www.amazon.com/Build-Amazing-After-Treatment-ebook/dp/B00G60UBLQ>.

[26] Woodbury, Debbie. *You Can Thrive After Treatment*, WhereWeGoNow, LLC, 2013. <http://www.amazon.com/You-Can-Thrive-After-Treatment-ebook/dp/B00EZWXXOY>.

[27] Sign up form, *The WhereWeGoNow Gratitude Gems Series: Your 30-Day Guide to Jump Starting a Lifetime Gratitude Practice*. Web. 29 Oct. 2013. <http://wherewegonow.us2.listmanage.com/subscribe?u=915e27d7085c84e5a4a24ef74&id=db818ecfb0>.

[28] Woodbury, Debbie collection of blog posts, The Huffington Post, Web. 29 Oct. 2013. < http://www.huffingtonpost.com/debbie-woodbury>.

[29] *Cancer Hope Network*, Web. 29 Oct. 2013. <http://www.cancerhopenetwork.org>.

[30] *Pathways Women's Cancer Teaching Project*. Web. 29 Oct. 2013. <http://womenscancerteachingproject.org/>.

[31] "Survivor Defined." Interview by Jennifer Gangloff. *Curetoday*. Cure Media Group, 16 Mar. 2013. Web. 29 Oct. 2013. <http://curetoday.com/index.cfm/fuseaction/journey.showArticle/id/9/enableStageSubMenu/5/article_id/2082>.

[32] "Seeing Red: Coping with Anger During Cancer." Interview by Heather L. Van Epps, Ph.D. *Curetoday*. Cure Media Group, 12 June 2012. Web. 29 Oct. 2013. <http://www.curetoday.com/index.cfm/fuseaction/article.show/id/2/article_id/1937>.

[33] Woodbury, Debbie. How to Build an Amazing Life After Treatment, WhereWeGoNow, LLC, 2013. <http://www.amazon.com/Build-Amazing-After-Treatment-ebook/dp/B00G60UBLQ>.

[34] Woodbury, Debbie on Twitter @DebbieWWGN, Web. 29 Oct. 2013. <https://twitter.com/DebbieWWGN>.

[35] WhereWeGoNow as Cancer Survivors, Facebook page. Web. 29 Oct. 2013 <https://www.facebook.com/pages/WhereWeGoNow-As-Cancer-Survivors/197760313589739>.

www.ingramcontent.com/pod-product-compliance
Lightning Source LLC
Chambersburg PA
CBHW070843290526
45795CB00002B/964